Why New Runners Fail: 26 Ultimate Tips You Should Know Before You Start Running!

by Scott Oscar Morton

All rights reserved. This book or parts thereof may not be reproduced in any form, stored in any retrieval system, or transmitted in any form by any means — electronic, mechanical, photocopy, recording, or otherwise — without prior written consent of the publisher, except as provided by United States of America copyright law. For reproduction rights, write to the publisher, at "Attention: Reproduction Rights," at the address below.

© 2017 by LERK Publishing, LLC. All rights reserved.

LERK Publishing, LLC.

Edited by Krystal Boots

Cover by LERK Publishing, LLC.

ISBN 978-1-947010-03-1
Edition 2.0

Follow me on Facebook and Twitter:

Twitter: @BeginR2FinishR

Facebook: facebook.com/BeginnerToFinisher/

Website: www.halfmarathonforbeginners.com

Email: scottmorton@halfmarathonforbeginners.com

To my wife Mieke.

Medical Disclaimer

The information in this book is meant to supplement, not replace, proper training. A sport involving speed, equipment, balance and environmental factors, and running, will involve some inherent risk. The authors and publisher advise readers to take full responsibility for their safety and know their limits. Before practicing the skills described in this book, be sure that your equipment is well maintained, and do not take risks beyond your level of experience, aptitude, training, and comfort level.

Why I Wrote This Book

I wrote this book for anyone with a burning desire to start running. The compilation of 26 reasons why beginning runners fail will hopefully steer you clear of common avoidable running mistakes. If I can help at least one person avert injury and pursue a hobby of running, then all the time put into this book will be worthwhile.

I designed this book for anyone with a desire to take up running to get in shape, to race competitively, or just to change up their exercise routine. This book is not intended to be a guide for experienced runners. However, there might very well be something that the experienced runner might learn from it.

I do hope this book keeps you running safe and injury free for years to come. The best of luck to you on your running path to success.

Injuries & Medical Conditions

If you have sports related injuries, I highly suggest that you talk to a medical professional to determine if you are fit enough to run. Not seeking medical advice could further exacerbate an existing injury. I am not a legal or medical professional, nor am I offering any type of legal or medical advice. One last time, if you're injured or have medical conditions that may prevent you from taking on a rigorous running training program, please seek the opinion of a licensed physician before participating in any physical training.

Other Books by Scott Oscar Morton

Sign up for FREE EBook releases of my new books at: http://geni.us/NRtsKu

Beginner to Finisher Series:

READ FOR FREE with Kindle Unlimited.

Available Now

Why New Runners Fail: 26 Ultimate Tips You Should Know Before You Start Running! Book 1 of 5
http://geni.us/WhyNewRunnersFail

5K Fury: 10 Proven Steps to Get You to the Finish Line in 9 weeks or less! Book 2 of 5
http://geni.us/5kFury

Beginner's Guide to Half Marathons: A Simple Step-By-Step Solution to Get You to the Finish line in 12 Weeks! Book 4 of 5
http://geni.us/HM4Beginners

Coming Soon

Beginner's Guide to 10Ks: A Simple Step-By-Step Solution to Get You to the Finish line in 9 Weeks! Book 3 of 5

Marathon Motivator: A Simple Step-By-Step Solution to get you to the Finish line in 20 Weeks! Book 5 of 5

Assumptions

Before you dive into this book, I'm assuming the following:

- You are new to running.
- You want tips to help you jump start your running career safely.
- You plan on sticking with running for the long term.

Reason #1
No self-motivation

Not being self-motivated will kill a runner's career before it even takes off. Being self-motivated ties into a much bigger scheme in the runner's mindset. If a runner's mind has not already committed to achieving a specific goal such as running a 5k, 10K, half marathon, or marathon, then you are running against yourself.

If you suffer from a lack of self-motivation, you can try out a few options. First, find a running partner. Running partners help keep you honest and motivate you to be somewhere to run. They keep you accountable. Running clubs could be a second place to look for motivation. They meet as often as once a week all the way up to once a month. Running clubs could be a better alternative to a running partner because running clubs tend to have more than two people as running partners. You can more easily find someone to run with that is more your style. The only problem with running clubs is that they might not meet as often as your running schedule, so you still have to have a little self-motivation to keep you going on the non-club meeting days.

Social media and online forums can also help keep you motivated. After you run a session or race, post your data to a forum or a social media site. People can comment on your running, giving you praise for your efforts.

Also, don't forget another motivator for running - losing weight. If you stick with running for at least four weeks and run at least three times a week, you will more than likely start losing weight. The key to losing weight is to not overeat beyond your daily caloric intake. Where new runners go wrong is thinking that they just ran 4 miles and burnt 600 calories so they can eat a cheeseburger. Well, this is true only if your surplus calories can offset the cost of the cheeseburger calories. The best way to do this is to count your calories using one of many calorie calculator apps. A few are Living Strong, Lose It!, My Fitness Pal, and many others.

Action steps:

- Find a running partner.
- Find a running club.
- Post your running data to forums or social media.
- Use the benefit of losing weight as a motivator.
- Use the benefit of being in better health.

Reason #2
Running when it's too hot outside

When you're new to running, you want to run whenever your schedule permits you to. While running in the cold just requires layering more clothes to keep your body warm, the heat requires fewer layers and more fluid. When the temperature starts extending into the 80's, your body has to work that much harder to sustain your running pace.

For example, let's pretend we make three identical copies of you and place them in three different environments.

- Runner 1 - runs in an environment below 40 degrees
- Runner 2 - runs in an environment between 50 degrees and 70 degrees
- Runner 3 - runs in an environment above 80 degrees

Which runner would sweat the most? The answer is obvious (Runner 3), yet many runners will run in the middle of July in Texas around 4 pm when temperatures get into the 100's and the heat index peaks around 110 degrees. Running in extreme temperatures does your body no service except for excess sweating and rapid fatigue. Even elite athletes shouldn't run in hot conditions.

Some critics think that running in extreme temperatures can help condition and strengthen the body. If you are an elite athlete that runs more than 50 miles a week, then running in hot environments can make you more resilient to extreme conditions. However, if you are an elite athlete, I seriously doubt you will be reading this book. For a beginner runner, you want to stack the odds in your favor by not running in hot temperatures.

Action steps:

- Run when the temperature is below 80 degrees.
- Run at night after the sun settles.
- Run indoors on a treadmill.
- Run in the morning before the sun rises above the horizon.

Reason #3
Not stretching before running

Do not perform static stretching before running. The only type of stretching needed before running is dynamic stretching. What is the difference between static and dynamic stretching? Static stretching movements performed correctly are stretches that require no active movement before doing the stretch. They are hold-and-release stretches, such as a standing quad stretch. Dynamic stretching is stretching with a continuous movement that is relative to your sports activity. An example of a dynamic stretch is walking knee raises where your body is continuously walking and you perform a set consisting of ten knee raises.

Your goal for pre-running stretching is it should take no longer than about ten minutes total. You can perform 4 or 5 different dynamic stretches and then jog lightly to warm-up. The real take away value is gained when you do some stretching or light running to warm up before you hit the multi-mile runs.

Action steps:

- Do not perform static stretching before running.
- Warm-up for a maximum of ten minutes with dynamic stretching.

Reason #4
Not stretching after running

Static stretching should be performed only after your core running training and after you have performed your cool down walk. Examples of static stretching range from a standing quad stretch to sitting advanced hurdler stretches.

The standing quad stretch is performed by standing on one leg and bending the knee of the other leg backward towards your rear end. Your arm should finish off the stretch by pulling your leg into your bottom as close as possible without causing pain. The exercise should feel a little uncomfortable but not painful. Hold for about ten to twenty seconds and then switch legs and repeat the stretch.

You perform the sitting advanced hurdler by sitting upright with one leg stretched out in front of you. Your other leg should be in a crossed perpendicular position pointing out from your current position. The crossed foot should lay flat touching the side of your other leg's inner knee. Use your arm on the same side as the leg that is stretched out in front of you and touch your toes. Lean your back over and try to touch your nose to your knee. The goal is not to try and touch your knee, but to give you something to lean into while you stretch.

The most important part of static stretching is not to bounce when you are stretching. The ideal form of static stretching is to hold and release, which should take anywhere from ten to twenty seconds for one stretch.

Action steps:

- Perform static stretching only after running, not before.
- Don't bounce during the stretch.
- Hold the stretch for ten to twenty seconds then release.

Reason #5
Running too fast too quickly

I see this on the running trail at least once a week. A beginner runner dashes by you, gasping for breath as they throw their legs out in front of them slamming their feet into the pavement over and over again. They might make it around the half-mile trail once, but after the first half-mile, they begin to crash. I have seen new runners almost fall over onto the ground. I've had to stop and ask runners if they were all right because it looked as if they passed out standing up. These runners appear most frequently after the start of a new year and about a month before swimsuit season. Let's make sure that you aren't one of these runners.

If you want to progress in the sport of running, you should have a training plan. I understand that some people just want to run for the sake of running, which is fine. However, if you channel those runs into a training plan, you will eventually become a better runner, almost guaranteed. Why? Because weekly training plans help push you a little bit each day and each week. Otherwise, you could end up plateauing your runs without any further progression. There are hundreds of free running training plans out there and even apps that help you on a daily and weekly basis.

If you are brand new to running, I suggest training for a 1-mile fun run race. Races usually have a kids run or fun run that anyone can join. Training your body to run one mile is not as hard as it looks. If a fun run sounds too childish, then you can train for a 5K. There are 5K races year round almost every weekend in cities all over the United States. Depending on your fitness level, you could be trained for a 5K in as little as four weeks.

Don't go out and run just yet. Finish reading this quick e-book before you start running. You will be glad you did.

Action steps:

- Don't go out and start running as fast as you can.
- A training plan will help your body slowly adjust to running.

Reason #6
No support system

Running can be a lonely sport. For some of us, we thrive on the solitude of the sport. No one to hold us back. I can run when I want to. For others, they need a social support system.

I fall into the category of not needing a social support system. In fact, my wife didn't know I had been training for a half marathon until about three weeks before my first race. My wife, on the other hand, needs social support to get motivated to work out. She finds it much easier for her to work out if she has an accountability partner or attends group workout sessions.

Many running apps allow you to set up your account for others to cheer you on during a run and give positive feedback in forums when you post your runs on-line. With platforms such as Instagram, you can add hashtags such as #Running or #BeginnerRunner and things of this nature that will allow others out there that you might not even know to give you positive feedback. Telling your work friends or your spouse that you are going to start running will also help you through continued encouragement.

There are also jogging clubs or meetups in cities all over the world that meet up in a group to share and be part of common interests, such as running.

Action steps:

- If you need support, look for apps that allow users and friends to cheer you on.
- Tell everyone you are starting to run.
- Find an accountability partner to help motivate you on bad days.
- Look for running meet-up groups.

Reason #7
Following incorrect training

If you are brand new to running, you need to start with a training program for beginners. You would think that most people would adhere to these words of wisdom, but think again. Most injuries from new runners happen as a result of incorrect training programs. This situation occurs when a new runner starts a beginner training program and follows one week's training successfully. Over the weekend they are zapped with delusions of grandeur and start looking up advanced training programs. The next week they implement the advanced training program. This training shortcut increases the likelihood of a sports running injury.

Another fallacy occurs when a new runner witnesses a veteran runner's race times and tries to train exactly like that person. The problem with this is that the veteran runner has run for years and years and knows the inner workings of a training program. A new runner can't follow a veteran's path immediately because they must build a strong weekly running base like the veteran did so that they can sustain a lifetime of running.

Action steps:

- Train at the level you are at.
- Training shortcuts don't exist, so don't take them.

Reason #8
Not enough rest

Sleep is essential to help fortify your running legs and replenish and repair your body. Just like anything else in life, if you want to be good at it, you have to be able to focus and concentrate on the subject at hand. Running or any other sports activity requires adequate rest to achieve any progress in the particular sport. When you couple lack of rest and drinking alcohol in the same period, you are multiplying the lack of sleep. Alcohol has been found to cause an interrupted sleep cycle. I'm not saying you need to abstain from drinking. Instead, don't drink on nights when you have to get up and run the following morning. Or if you do drink, allow yourself only two drinks for the evening.

If you run long distances once a week, you should allow yourself a one day break after your run session. The 24 hours following a long distance run should be used primarily for resting and rebuilding your muscles so that they can increase your glycogen stores to allow you to fuel your body for longer runs. Skipping this rest day does not give your body enough time to repair itself between runs.

If you are planning on running a half marathon or marathon, I suggest you take a look at my book *Beginner's Guide to Half Marathons*.

Action steps:

- Get at least 7 to 8 hours sleep a night before a run day.
- Allow 1 day to rest after a long duration run (excess of 6 miles).

Reason #9
Running too little

Running too little will not allow your body to get used to a training schedule. For example, let's say that you only run two days a week—let's pick Monday and Thursday–to run. Each session consists of 1 mile running followed by 1 mile of walking.

Negatives:
- Your body isn't getting used to running.
- You might be more susceptible to injury because your body isn't able to rebuild and reuse the muscles quickly enough. It's almost like your body is forgetting how to run between workouts.
- You won't be able to progress much further than your training mileage.
- Inadequate running makes the mental struggle harder on the mind. Your mind and body think they are being reset after each run session and are not learning the habit of running.

Positives:
- You are exercising.

I don't think that you should ever drop below an absolute minimum of three days running/walking. I prefer at least four days of running. If you decide to run a maximum of three days, I highly suggest that you skip every other day (see below).

Three days of training

Mon.	Tues.	Wed.	Thur.	Fri.	Sat.	Sun.
Run	Rest	Run	Rest	Run	Rest	Walk

Four days of training (Preferred)

Mon.	Tues.	Wed.	Thur.	Fri.	Sat.	Sun.
Run	Run	Rest	Run	Rest	Run	Walk

Action steps:

- Running too little makes it tougher on your body than having a normal running schedule.
- Don't run less than 3 times a week if you want to progress in the sport of running.

Reason #10
Running too often

The more days a week you run as a beginner, the quicker your body will fall to fatigue and the more likely you will give up running for the rest of your life. I don't want this to happen to you.

Pick three days as a minimum amount of days to run for a week. It's best not to stack your running days such as Monday, Tuesday, and Wednesday. There is too long of a gap between Wednesday and next Monday. It's better to stagger the running days like Monday-Run, Tuesday-off, etc.

I don't recommend running 5+ days a week unless you are a seasoned runner. The more days of the week you are running, the less time the body has to repair itself. If you are a beginner runner, your body hasn't molded itself into a "runner's body" yet. The seasoned runner has already been sculpted into a lean mean running machine. A revved up body is possible through habitually running on a weekly basis and years of repetitive sessions.

Action steps:

- Pick 3-4 days of the week to run; rest or cross train on the remaining days.

Reason #11
Wrong socks and shoes

I learned the hard way about socks and shoes. When I began running, I threw on a pair of no-show white socks and a pair of $50 "running" shoes I found at Academy Sports. I was excited about getting to the gym and giving my new shoes a spin. I ran in the shoes for about three days. At the end of my run session on the third day, I felt a pain in the back of my heel. I took off my sock and noticed a large red blister the size of a quarter. The blister appeared as a result of cheaply made no-show socks and the incorrect "running" shoes I purchased.

If you are serious about running, don't make the mistake that I did and buy cheaply designed socks and shoes. You can buy a good pair of running shoes for a minimum of $80, and you can spend as much as $160 on elite running shoes. I choose Nike because they offer a free return on shoes purchased within 30 days if you tried them out and didn't like them. The ultimate choice for me was the Nike Free RN shoes. These shoes offer lots of support, especially for runners that weigh 200+ pounds, which is me.

The best running shoe varies between motion-controlled, cushioned, and stabilized. How do you know what type of shoe you need? The simple answer is travel to your local running store and let them test you on a machine that shows your foots pronation in the gait cycle. Pronation comes down to how well your foot absorbs shock from each cycle during running.

Action steps:

- Buy a good pair of running shoes. Just like all sports, there are small investments that are required.
- Buy at least two pairs of descent running socks that prevent blistering.
- If you buy running shoes and they hurt your feet or legs, take a trip to your local running store to check gait cycle (pronation).

Reason #12
Following running trends without research

The Internet is a tidal wave of information. There are tons of free resources floating around about running, including training schedules, methods of running, how many days a week you should run, and so forth. Before you buy into a new training system, check to make sure the system is proven. Also, make sure that it's for the right type of runner. There are several different types of runners, including beginners, intermediate, advanced, and elite runners. Be wary of training plans that state you will get a personal best run time for your first half marathon if you follow their system. Some elite runners in the field have been running for years to beat their personal best records.

Action steps:

- Watch out for outlandish claims from beginning training systems.
- Try to find logically safe, proven training systems.

Reason #13
Poor Dieting

We've all heard the same information over and over again about eating a balanced diet. We all need to lose weight, and we all want to have a lean, athletic body. Runners, of all people, should know the difference between eating a healthy meal and a nutritionally starved meal, right?

You slap on your Garmin, Fitbit, Apple Watch, or whatever techno device to start tracking those steps and miles. You run for a good 5 miles at a decent pace and work up a sweat. You slow down to a walking pace to enter your cool down phase. You sync your device to the phone, and you stare in amazement when your tracking app shows you that your body burned 500+ calories. (This is assuming that you burn 100 calories a mile. For larger framed beginner runners, your calorie per mile consumption can be as high as 175 calories a mile. The 100 calories per mile is an average of all runners. See the section on burning calories for a more in depth discussion.)

Your mind begins to throw images of what kinds of food you can eat with the surplus of calories. Instead of replacing the 500 calorie surplus with good food, new runners tend to go for the burger or side of fries. While there is nothing wrong with a burger and fries every once in a while, the problem lies with the fact that the nutritional value you get from these foods is less than what you would have gotten from a lean meat followed by fruits and vegetables. Boring, right? Elite runners have known this for a long time. What you eat directly affects your performance while running.

Some nutritional guides will tell you that you should never eat processed foods and when you have one cheat day where you can eat whatever you want to, your body takes at least a few weeks before recovering from the surge of non-nutritional food. I'm not asking you to go crazy hardcore with your diet. Instead, be mindful and try to choose better foods for your body.

Action steps:

- Limit intake of fast foods and processed foods.
- Limit fried food consumption.
- If you do have an "eat anything" day, try to make it on the weekend and don't overdo it.

Reason #14
Over racing

Once you've finished a race, congratulate yourself on completing the race. Take a few extra days to rest. If it's your first finished race, you need to take extra time to rest and relax. There are runners out there that run a half marathon every two weeks, and some elite runners run twelve plus marathons a year. These elite runners are such a super small sect of runners that you have to call them elite runners. For the average runner, you should only compete in a maximum of two marathons a year. Is it possible to do more? Of course, but at what cost to your body?

Running a 5k race every weekend is doable, but I don't even suggest doing that until you are a more seasoned runner. How long until you can start running more races? I would run at least an entire year before starting to attempt multiple races during one calendar month. If you are a younger runner, then you might already be well acclimated to running multiple races a month.

Listening to your body and knowing its limitations is one of the most important rules for runners. Rest is probably more important than the actual running for new runners. Without consistent repair of the body after running sessions, your body will never fully heal, and you won't reach your full potential as a new runner.

Action steps:

- Limit 5K and 10K races to no more than one a month.
- Limit your half marathon races to no more than one every three months (four a year total).
- Limit your marathons to no more than one every six months (twice a year total).

Reason #15
Not listening to your body

"Listen to your body" in running terms is simpler than it sounds. When you begin running, listening to your body isn't realistic until you are running 2 miles or greater in a run session. Listening to your body allows you to interrupt any tangents your mind might be racing off to while running. I'm not proposing that you shut off the flow of information in your head, but there may be times when your body starts to stiffen up or your breathing is off. I go through a set of techniques to help my running form if I feel my body just letting go.

    1) I make sure my head is upright and my back is leaning slightly forward. Do not tuck your head into your chest. If you tuck your head into your chest, correct this quickly as this could lead to a lot of aches and pains.

    2) Make sure you're breathing in and out of both your nose and mouth. If you are gasping for air, your body is more than likely fatigued or you're working your body too hard.

    3) If you are struggling with breathing, try to create a breath-step cycle. A breath-step cycle is running a certain amount of steps per one breath. For example, when you're running, start counting the steps after you have breathed out. Breathe in slowly while counting your steps, then exhale slowly counting your steps. Your breath cycle should be anywhere between 10 and 20 steps. My breath-step cycle is 12 steps per one breath. If you practice doing this over and over again, it will become natural, and you will feel more in control of your breathing.

Action steps:

- Breathe in and out while running and count your steps.
- When you feel your form slacking, remember your breath-step count and track them in your head.
- If you are tensing up, relax your shoulders.
- If you are tightening up while running, slow down to a walk and stretch.

Reason #16
Running while injured

Running while injured is probably the worst thing a beginner runner or any runner could do. For example, let's say you bought a cheap pair of running shoes and ran for about a week in them. The following week your shins and knees start hurting in places they have never hurt before. Your body is sending out signals of pain telling you that you need to fix something involving your feet or legs. In most cases of new runners complaining about their feet hurting after running, it's almost always because of shoes. The only other reasons would be some debilitating leg disorder or prior leg injuries. Regardless, take a minimum of three days off from running and get your running feet checked out. Also, see if your shoes match which pronation your feet tend to use during their run cycle (see the wrong socks and shoe section).

Action steps:

- If your feet or shins hurt, check your shoes.
- If you experience any pain treat with caution. Usually two to three days of no running will help alleviate the pain.
- If you suspect that your shoes are causing you pain, visit your local running store, and bring your running shoes with you.

Reason #17
Running without cross training

Have you ever seen the elite runners with great-looking, muscular legs, but then the camera pans up to show they have the meekest body? It happens a lot. While not cross-training your upper body doesn't affect a runner's performance, it does affect your appearance. It's the same for weight trainers that concentrate most of their efforts on lifting with the upper body and spend less time with the trunk and legs. Sometimes people will describe weight trainers that fit that appearance as having "chicken" legs.

Weight resistance training, walking, biking, and yoga are all sources of terrific cross-training. You should avoid stair steppers when you are training for long distance races over 5 miles. Stair steppers activate different parts of the leg muscles.

Cross-training also helps with overall blood circulation of the body and turning more of your body fat into muscle.

Action steps:

- Don't just run; try to mix in at least one day of full body weight training.
- If you don't choose to weight train, consider at least yoga, extra walking, or bicycling.

Reason #18
Breathing patterns

If you have meditated before, you have heard the terminology "follow your breath" and "just breathe in and breathe out." Breath is no more than a systematic response to the body exhaling unneeded carbon dioxide and breathing in the much-needed oxygen. Since breathing is innate to every human born, it makes sense to follow breathing patterns when we run.

When we run, the mind and body move more smoothly if they lock into a pattern that allows ultimate efficiency. If you run with short breaths while you're training, you're robbing your body of much-needed oxygen and energy. A shallow breath runner will always run slower and less efficiently than a deep breather, also known as bottom breathing (breathing into the bottom portion of the lungs). When a runner exhibits short breaths, it's indicative of inefficient breathing or running fatigue.

Breathing Cadence

If you practice this simple example, your breathing should improve almost immediately when you run. The key is to breathe in while running three strides and breathe out while running another three strides. This pattern is known as breathing cadence. Using this technique will help refocus your efforts on running and breathing in a state of flow, which will help relax the body, causing it to run more efficiently.

The difference between a stride and a step is defined as a step being only one foot striking the ground and a stride is both the left and right feet striking the ground. To practice breathing cadence while running, count the number of times one of your feet strikes the ground while inhaling and then count the number of times while exhaling.

What you will find is that you will have one of the following ratios:

Inhale Strides	Exhale Strides	Ratio
2	2	2:2
3	3	3:3

Breathing Cadence of a 2:2 ratio tells you you are breathing a little quicker and shallower. While, a 3:3 ratio tells you that you are breathing a little slower with deeper breaths. Some runners will have 3:2 ratio which might be normal for their running style.

If you count your strides for 15 seconds and multiply by 4 this will give you your running cadence. Your running cadence, also called your stride rate, should be somewhere at or above 120 strides per minutes. An average running cadence is around 160. For a beginner runner, this number doesn't hold much water, however counting your strides while running will help normalize your breathing during runs. Elite runners strive to achieve a cadence of 180 plus. Can you still be an efficient runner and breathe shallow? Yes, however, you could be a more efficient runner if you focused on taking deeper breaths.

If you have trouble tracking your breathing cadence while running, don't sweat it. Overall it will have a marginal impact on your overall performance. Your running posture, pace, not over striding, and hydration, play much bigger roles in your overall performance. Another solution would be to try out yoga. At its core, yoga strives for breathing efficiency by holding poses coupled with steady, deep breathing.

Action steps:

- Stop shallow breathing when running (i.e. huffing and puffing).
- Focus on deep breathing when running.
- If you have trouble deep breathing while running, do some Yoga.

Reason #19
Running posture

Running Posture

Your running posture is just as important as breathing correctly. Before I dive into what good running posture looks like, let's explore what your posture shouldn't model.

Incorrect running posture:
- Bouncing when running - springs in your step cause irregular fatigue in your muscle when you land.
- Running standing straight up - your body will not be able to endure long runs if your back is straight up.
- Running with tense shoulders - relax your shoulders.
- Running with arms fully extended in both directions - your arms should bend no more than 120 degrees downward.
- Running with your arms packed tightly next to the chest - you are wasting energy keeping your arms tense and tucked next to your chest.
- Allowing your feet to run in front of you - unless you are purposely sprinting.

Correct Running Posture:
- Your feet should land right in front of your legs.
- Your feet should glide heel to toe, step after step.
- Your back should be slightly bent forward.
- Your shoulders should be pressed backward but without tension.
- Your entire body should lean slightly forward, almost like your body is about to fall but not quite.
- Your arms naturally swing forward.
- You're breathing deeply.
- Run with smaller steps.

Action steps:

- Don't run with a rigid back; always lean slightly forward when running.
- If you focus on correcting your breathing, all of the other postures issues should naturally correct themselves.

Reason #20
Vertical oscillation - don't bounce

What is vertical oscillation? If you think of an oscillating floor fan, the fan goes back and forth from one extent to another. When running, your feet follow a cycle and have a peak and a valley when they run (high point and low point). Vertical oscillation is the measure of how much bounce is in your step. The less bounce you have in your step, the less oscillation and the faster you will run. Why is this the case? If you look at elite track runners, you will notice that not one of them is bouncing while they are running. Each bounce has a double negative impact. The first negative impact is on your time. When your foot springs up rather than glides horizontally across the ground, it takes more time to reach the ground from your bounce. Secondly, if your running step has bounce, you increase the likelihood of a foot injury. Your landing foot has to cushion more impact from your body being higher in the air. It's not that each bounce impacts your body as much as it is the totality of 100 or 1,000 cushioned impacted steps that wear out and harm your feet.

Action steps:

- Don't bounce when you run.
- Try to make your body glide from step to step by concentrating on your legs pulling you forward instead of pushing you forward.

Reason #21
Not knowing what to do next

Not knowing what to do next can kill your running career before you even begin. For a new runner, it's hard to know exactly just how far to take your running career. I suggest starting off slow and signing up for a 5k race at least eight to six weeks out. This time frame will give you a lot of time to get you from zero running to 3.1 miles within an eight week period. I hear some of you groaning right now, and I will give you this piece of advice - running is as much mental as it is a physical sport. Impossible! The truth is that running takes as much mental focus and motivation as the exhausting physical aspect of running. If you start your 5k training with a negative mental attitude such as "I will never be able to finish a 5K," then it will resonate throughout your training. One of the easiest ways to get around these negative attitudes is telling yourself every morning and every night that you are training for a 5K. The secret word in that sentence is "training." When you use "training" and not "workout," your body switches itself into a wanting to do mode rather than a having to do mode. I want to train for my 5K so I can finish. I have to work out so that I will lose weight. The difference is slight yet powerful.

Action steps:

- Don't run for the sake of running unless you are extremely self-motivated.
- Sign up for a 5K and at the least start scheduling your runs once a week. This will help plant the seeds in your head that you will be running a certain amount of days for the upcoming week.

Reason #22
Completely stopping following a run

After any running session lasting more than a mile, you should keep moving even after you stop running. Your muscles need to cool down, which is the start of the recovery cycle. Many runners suggest walking between ten and twenty minutes depending on how many miles you ran. Others use distance instead of a time interval for cooling down. I find it more useful to use a cool down walking distance. Below are the minimum distances I walk based on how many miles I ran for a given run session.

Miles Ran	Cool down (miles)	Cool down (minutes)
0 - 4	1/2	10
4 - 10	1	20
10 +	1 1/2	30

Choosing either a timed cooldown or a distance cooldown will reduce injury and help your recovery cycle. Feel free to walk longer or for a greater length of time; doing so will help you burn extra calories and ensure your body is properly cooled down.

Action steps:

- Your cool down time should be no shorter than 10 minutes for any given run.
- Choose to use either a time interval or distance for cooldowns.

Reason #23
Not staying hydrated

You would think that hydration would be an easy one for runners to tackle. We've all heard the saying about each person needing to drink at least 64 oz of water a day, which equates to eight, 8 oz glasses a day. How does being a runner and sweating excessively change things for hydration? Not much. Your body still needs a baseline of fluids that starts at around 64 oz of water.

Three things that runners need to heed when dealing with hydration issues are hot running environments, dehydration due to excessive alcohol consumption, and fluids lost during a run session.

Running during hot temperatures forces your body to increase sweat to cool the body down, resulting in extra energy wasted. Hot temperatures require you to hydrate more often than in colder temperatures.

Running the next day after excessive alcohol consumption puts your hydration level at another risk. Before you start running, your body is under-hydrated due to your body fighting off the alcohol. Even if you use the rule of one eight ounce water per one twelve ounce beer, you still run the risk of being under-hydrated. I use the general rule of thinking before drinking. If I know that my running schedule shows me that I need to run more than 3 miles the next day, I drink a maximum of two drinks. If my schedule calls for running four miles plus, I don't drink at all. A runner's age also plays a big role when dealing with alcohol and running. A runner in their early twenties can recover easier than someone in their thirties or forties. If you want to become an elite runner, then alcohol needs to be taken out of the entire training cycle, or you won't become elite.

Lastly, the fluid weight you lose during runs needs to be replenished. How do you figure out how much fluid you lost during a run? Weigh yourself with all of your gear on before you run and write the number down. After your run, dry off and weigh yourself again with the same gear you had on. The difference in weight is the amount of fluid you lost during a run. For my half marathon race, I lost four pounds of fluids, which is approximately 64 ounces of water. Some runners lose up to six to eight pounds during a race. The normal amount of fluid lost should be anywhere between 0.25 pound to four pounds for runs under ten miles. In cooler weather, you will probably sweat less and not lose as much weight when compared to hotter weather.

How do you tell if you are under-hydrated, hydrated, or over-hydrated? The easiest way is to examine the color of your urine. Clear urine is a sign that you're over-hydrated. A light yellow to a pale lemonade color is hydrated. A darker apple juice color indicates your body is under-hydrated.

Action steps:

- Drink plenty of water, especially during your training.
- Don't run when it's too hot, but if you do wear a hydration pack.
- Check your urine to see how hydrated you are.

Reason #24
Not scheduling your runs

Most people who run long term get a sense of enrichment out of it, such as health, cardio, appearance, or achievement benefits. If you want to make sure that you are holding yourself accountable for your weekly runs, try scheduling your runs out for the week on Sunday. For me, Sunday is my rest day. I don't run or cross-train at all on Sundays. If I do any exercise at all on Sunday, I will walk for a few miles.

Grab your calendar or runner's log and schedule out your runs (click here to get a runner's log). For a new runner, I would recommend running no more than 2-3 times a week staggered until you are getting used to running. Your body needs to adjust to running slowly. Don't forget that you can approach running with a walk-run method where you walk for 3 minutes and then run for 3 minutes and switch back and forth for a mile or two. Some new runners might want to put more emphasis on walking than running until they have adjusted their bodies. An example would be to walk 4 minutes and run 1 minute then repeat.

I am going to assume that you can walk the distance of 1 mile. A good test to determine what runner level you are at is to first walk the distance of a mile. Time your walk and write it down. After you have walked a mile (consider this your warm-up), attempt to run for one mile. If you know you are unable to run the distance of one mile now, that's OK. It's OK if you are huffing and puffing, but remember the reason for listening to your body. Your body is telling you that you are fatigued and can't run the 1 mile.

I suggest running 1 mile 2-3 times a week to start off with and progress from there.

<u>Can't run 1 mile</u>
Walk for 5 minutes; run for 1 minute (repeat)

<u>Can run 1 mile but difficult</u>
Walk for 4 minutes; run for 1 minute (repeat)

<u>Can run 1 mile but not too difficult</u>
Walk for 3 minutes; run for 1 minute (repeat)

<u>Can run 1 mile easily</u>
Walk for 2 minutes; run for 2 minutes (repeat)

<u>Can run 1 mile super easy</u>
Walk for 1 minute; run for 3 minutes (repeat)

Action steps:

- Schedule your runs once a week for the upcoming week.
- Stick to your schedule; if you can't run in the morning try running in the evening.
- Determine how far you can run without walking up to the distance of a mile to help schedule your running sessions.

Reason #25
Plateauing

As a new runner, you don't have to worry about plateauing immediately, but it's a good thing to go ahead and plant the seed. Plateauing is just as it sounds. If you picture a plateau as you drive along through the desert, you can observe how the top of a mountain looks like it was evenly chopped off making it look flat. Plateauing can happen in anything in life such as work, diets, and of course running. When we start out our new running career, we are constantly building from a base mileage, requiring us to train our legs, body, and mind to become more efficient runners.

If you ran 1 mile 3 times a week for a year, your body would become super-efficient at conquering one mile. Once you obtain your goal of 3.1 miles, for example, you can continuously get better at 3.1 miles, and maybe that's all you want to do. The bigger picture I'm aiming at is to let you realize that sometimes it's important to change things up in your running cycle.

Below is an example of how you can change your running patterns and behavior so that you trick your body into triggering what I call runner resets. Runner resets will not erase all of your running mileage; it simply gives your legs a change in routine, which also allows your mind to trigger resets in the same way your physical body does.

1) Change your running route.

2) If you run an all flat course, add hills to your course.

3) Once per week you can do hill sprints, which is running up short hills multiple times in one session.

4) Run speed work drills, which involve interval training.

5) If you have the ability, run in a different geographic environment.

6) Run on trails instead of pavement.

7) Run in the sand on the beach.

8) Run random distances to various objects in a park.

9) Run on a track (once around is a quarter mile).

Action steps:

- Change up your running routine, especially if you feel yourself getting bored.
- Take a few extra days off if you're just not feeling it; then get back into it full-heartedly.

Reason #26
Not sticking with it

Running, like any other sport or activity you participate in, takes some time getting used to. When we were younger, we didn't have to think as much about running. We all looked forward to recess time at school. We would head outside and jump, hula hoop, walk and run without any conscious thought at all. Over the years, after finishing high school and possibly completing college, we ended up sitting on our rumps in a desk chair for extended periods of time. I have heard the excuses such as, "I don't have the genes to do it," or "You make running look easy." While some people can't physically run due to physical limitations or medical conditions, the rest of us don't have an excuse.

I ran my first 5k race when I was 37 years old with no training at all, which goes against one of my reasons why new runners fail - doing too much too fast. After my first 5K, I told myself that I would never run again. Never say never. After the 5K I thought deeply about me running the race and realized that I could have injured myself such as tearing an ACL or pulling hamstring muscles. Five years later I did the same thing again, no training, and I ran in another 5k race. I think that I actually should have got injured from lack of brains. But I didn't get injured. Instead, this set me off on a new path to running and figuring out as much as I could about the sport of running. I was able to race a 5k with no training and get second place in my age group. Was I lucky? You bet, but just showing up sometimes is half the battle of the race.

If you follow the guidelines in this book and start off slowly while at the same time listening to your body, you should be able to craft a running hobby or career that can take you as far as your legs will let you. Are you going to ache from time to time? Yes. Are there going to be days that you don't feel like running? Yes. Are there days that you will want to quit halfway through training for a particular race like a half marathon? More than certainly. How do you deal when your mind is being bombarded with thoughts like these? You have to push past it. Tell your body that you are just going to run for one mile. When you get out there and start running, your body will start to release endorphins that help mask the pain.

Action steps:

- Give running at least four weeks before thinking about quitting.
- Running has no shortcuts; you have to put in the time to get better.
- All elite runners were beginner runners at some point in time.
- Reward yourself for running your first mile.

Bonus #1
Extra Running Benefits

Extra benefits that come along with running are the obvious such as weight loss and getting in better shape.

Jogger's high is another advantage that some runners experience, while others have yet to experience it. It's a hit or miss experience. I have spoken with some runners that have never experienced jogger's high and have run for years. On the other hand, I have known runners that have only been running for a few months who have experienced a jogger's high. Jogger's high is overrated if you ask me. Your body gets a rush of euphoria, and you feel light and on top of the world, and you feel like you can run forever. The effect wears off quickly, probably within a few minutes, and it's back to normal running.

Some runners experience deep meditation while running. Runners claim to do their best thinking and most creative thinking while running. While running, if you focus on your breath like one of the reasons in this book, your body can reach a state of meditation. I have experienced a meditative state while running, but it takes great focus. This is when your body starts thinking about other things, and you forget you are running. Your legs and body are on autopilot, and you are still running. It sounds kind of hokey, but some runners, including myself, have experienced it so often.

Endorphins are another natural pain killer that your body releases while exercising, especially when running. For instance, your calf muscles may ache before running, but after a few miles of running your calf muscles should loosen up. In fact, just exercising in general for thirty minutes a day releases endorphins which in turn makes you a happier person.

Some scientists are now looking into possibilities that rigorous exercising might also help retrain the brain to loosen addictive behaviors and rewrite the neurons with more productive addictions such as exercise.

Bonus #2
Training Schedules for Absolute Beginners

There are 5280 feet in a mile, and the tables below show that if you start from 1 mile a week running and just slightly increase your running distance by 10% each week, you will reach the distance of a 5K, which is 3.1 miles in 13 weeks.

For Example:
Week 1 starts at 1.0 mile each day since this is the beginning of your training cycle; 0 additional miles are added the first week.

Week 2 adds 10% of Week 1's total miles, which is 1.1 miles per each day ran (1.0 miles + 0.1 miles = 1.1 miles).

Week #	Total Miles	Additional Miles
1	1.0	0
2	1.1	0.1
3	1.2	0.1
4	1.3	0.1
5	1.5	0.1
6	1.6	0.1
7	1.8	0.2
8	1.9	0.2
9	2.1	0.2
10	2.4	0.2
11	2.6	0.2
12	2.9	0.3
13	3.1	

If you increase your running distance by 20% each week, you will get to the distance of a 5k in about seven weeks.

Week #	Total Miles	Additional Miles
1	1.0	0
2	1.2	0.2
3	1.4	0.2
4	1.7	0.3
5	2.1	0.3
6	2.5	0.4
7	3.0	

If you increase your running distance by 30% each week, you will get to the distance of a 5k in about 5.5 weeks. As you can see, there is little difference between getting to the 3.1-mile goal by using a 20% increase versus a 30% increase. The biggest exception, if any, is with a 30% increase you would be running 3.7 miles.

Week #	Total Miles	Additional Miles
1	1.0	0
2	1.3	0.3
3	1.7	0.4
4	2.2	0.5
5	2.9	0.7
6	3.7	

Congratulations

Pat yourself on the back if you've started a running training program. No matter how long it takes you to reach your running goals, remember that while you are out there getting some miles in and helping yourself build a happier, healthier life, others are sitting on the couch watching TV or surfing on the Internet. Don't get discouraged if you have a bad day and a lousy run. Horrible runs happen to the best of runners. The key ingredient is to shake off the run. Verbally tell yourself that "This is no big deal," and get yourself out and running the next day. If you start harping on yourself for a lousy run, you are giving your mind and body an excuse to give up and quit. I don't want you to quit running because of one bad run. On my way to training for a half marathon and a marathon, I had several bad runs. In fact, during one of my ten mile runs during a half marathon training I had to stop running and vomited in a trash can. This bad run was entirely preventable by simply not drinking the night before a long duration run.

I'm illustrating this to you to show you that even marathon runners have bad runs. It happens, so get over it.

If I have to leave you with the best piece of advice for a long term running career, I give you this:

Resilience is what you need to get to the finish lines and beyond.

What's next?

If you want to continue your running career, I urge you to sign up for a 5K. If you are not interested in entering races, then try to maintain running a few times a week. I started out running 5Ks and didn't even consider myself a good enough runner to finish a marathon. But it turns out that I am a good enough runner, and you are too. The path to the longer races isn't an easy road, but if you stick with it and keep learning each week, finishing half marathons and marathons is attainable for average runners.

Other Books by Scott Oscar Morton

Sign up for FREE EBook releases of my new books at: http://geni.us/NRtsKu

Beginner to Finisher Series:

READ FOR FREE with Kindle Unlimited.

Available Now

Why New Runners Fail: 26 Ultimate Tips You Should Know Before You Start Running! Book 1 of 5
http://geni.us/WhyNewRunnersFail

5K Fury: 10 Proven Steps to Get You to the Finish Line in 9 weeks or less! Book 2 of 5
http://geni.us/5kFury

Beginner's Guide to Half Marathons: A Simple Step-By-Step Solution to Get You to the Finish line in 12 Weeks! Book 4 of 5
http://geni.us/HM4Beginners

Coming Soon

Beginner's Guide to 10Ks: A Simple Step-By-Step Solution to Get You to the Finish line in 9 Weeks! Book 3 of 5

Marathon Motivator: A Simple Step-By-Step Solution to get you to the Finish line in 20 Weeks! Book 5 of 5

About the Author

I played sports throughout my youth and even into my adult years. I ran my first 5k at the age of 37 in March of 2008 without any training at all. I finished in third place, although my leg muscles felt like I deserved first place. My legs were sore for six days after the race. My next 5k attempt was in 2015 at the age of 42 in my local hometown. I had no intention of placing at all. I ended up running worse than my first 5k by almost two minutes. I placed second with no training at all. I thought I would have learned a lesson by now - nope.

In May 2016, I was flying to Las Vegas for our yearly guys' trip. I was reading a Sky Mall magazine, and I came across an article called "Top 100 things to do in Las Vegas." Number eight on the list was run a race through the streets of Las Vegas. During the race, the city blocks off sections of the strip. I was hooked. They offered a 5k, 10k, half marathon and marathon. I liked walking a lot; in fact, one of my favorite things to do in Las Vegas was to see how many steps I could get in a day (my record to date is 42,000). The Rock-and-Roll Half Marathon/Marathon would be taking place in November 2016. I scoured the Internet for any information related to training for a half marathon.

My wife asked me, "Why in the world do you want to run a half marathon?" I told her because I was physically able to. She said, "You just want to put one of those 13.1 stickers on the back of your car." But truthfully the real reason was much deeper than that. Whenever I catch a fresh dump of powder on my snowboard, there is no other experience like it. I feel like a kid again, and I feel alive. The real reason I wanted to run was because I wanted to feel the accomplishment, feel the pain and feel the glory of crossing the finish line all the while feeling alive. Running allows me to unleash that competitive kid inside me which yearns to feel alive.

Help an Author Out

Thanks for reading! If you've enjoyed this book, please let me know how I can make this book better. Other shoppers on Amazon rely on ratings so that it can save them valuable time when shopping for new Ebooks. I take the time to read every review so that I can change and update this book based on reviewer feedback. Please go here to review the book:

http://geni.us/okn1Yr

If you've just finished a race and you want someone to tell, send me an email. I would be delighted to hear from you.

Follow me on Facebook and Twitter:

Twitter: @BeginR2FinishR

Facebook: facebook.com/BeginnerToFinisher/

Website: www.halfmarathonforbeginners.com

Email: scottmorton@halfmarathonforbeginners.com